Crossfit Training

Complete Guide On Healthy Eating And Home-cooked
Meal Plans For Weight Loss And Muscle Gain.

(Kettlebell Workouts For A Ripped Physique)

Deshawn Lambert

TABLE OF CONTENT

Know What You Want

You must first understand why you choose to go to the gym in the first place before you can ever consider going there.

Additionally, make sure your "WHY" is BIG and CLEAR.

Because your "WHY" is what motivates you to devote the most important resource you possess—your time—to this endeavor.

You don't always need a large one; it might be as simple as:

Desiring a positive atmosphere around oneself.
• Desiring to make NEW, POSITIVE friends.
Learning about something called Crossfit.
Adding value to your idle time.

Building strength and fitness.
Seeing your friends and enjoying yourselves.
- ...

What important is that you have a WHY, regardless of what that may be.

The most crucial factor in this situation is that you must make it about you.

For instance, if you're practicing Crossfit (lifting big weights, disobeying your coach, not paying attention to your warm-up or mobility exercises, etc.) in order to upload a video on Instagram (so you can flex.), prove to others that you can do a handstand, or if you can lift 350 kg in a back squat... You're screwed.

You are a Fucking IDIOT in my eyes.

First of all, since everyone has their own problems, no one cares about your sh*t.(They could be briefly impressed, but they'll soon forget...)

Second, you are simply attracting other FAKE individuals who are just like you.

You're reading this book, so I know you're not one of those folks. Reflect on it

A false person won't spend their time learning about the mindset of a Crossfit athlete because deep down they know that's not why they are at the gym.

Therefore, he or she is not required to understand what a Crossfit athlete is.

Doing what makes you HAPPY is the objective...

I'm your number one supporter on this whether posting videos on Instagram "for you" is to educate others or simply to share it.

To have a purpose for what you're doing at the gym, you need to know what your "WHY" is.

Remember: If you don't know where you're going, you won't get there.

What Constitutes a Good Meat Diet?

Here are some guidelines for a healthy craft diet:

fulfills your caloric needs

If you regularly work out at the gym, you will need to consume more calories than the average person. Inadequate calorie intake may initially result in weight reduction, but it will ultimately cause a plateau and a decrease in energy.

Optimal macronutrient intake

Consider balancing your carbohydrate, protein, and fat consumption until you get a balance that improves performance.

Adequate consumption of nutrients

essential vitamins and minerals that support your body's function and wellbeing.

according to your objectives

Depending on your expertise and objectives, your diet should account for what you'd want to achieve (such as weight loss, improved performance,

etc.). qualify for a certain CrossFit competition, etc.)
Balanced in a manner that promotes longevity
You will find eating to be a dreadful experience if you don't adopt a nutritional approach that takes into account your lifestyle and opportunities to "reap the rewards" of your fitness. This makes long-term health and fitness difficult to achieve. A healthy diet allows for occasional indulgences and delicious meals as well as days off.

How Do Macronutrients Work?
The fundamental components of all human diet are macronutrients. A Cro-Fitter needs an equal distribution of macros to fuel their efforts and recover properly.
There are three macronutrients: protein, carbohydrates, and fats. One gram of protein or carbohydrate has four calories, but one gram of fat contains nine.
The real building components of your diet are proteins. They aid in muscular

growth, hair growth, and the regulation of several bodily functions.

In the diet industry, carbohydrates have a bad rap. If you've ever followed a low-carb diet, you're probably already trained to despise them. Carbohydrates, however, fuel our efforts. The body converts carbohydrates into glucose so that we have the energy to do activities. Managing your carbohydrate intake with wise sources and careful consumption will help you get the most out of this remarkable tool for performance.

In our bodies, fat controls a variety of hormonal processes and maintains the health of our nervous system.

Although their caloric value never varies, not all macronutrients are produced equally. For instance, monounsaturated and polyunsaturated fats are regarded as the "healthy fat" because they include omega-3 fatty acids. Trans fats are not naturally occurring and are linked to several health concerns. Although saturated fat is sometimes seen negatively, it really depends on the source. Consuming saturated fat from an organic egg is not the same as doing so from a Twizzler. In any case, they are entirely fat, which means they have 9 calories per gram.

What Are Micronuclei?

A healthy body need micronutrients, such as vitamins and minerals, to operate properly. They are necessary for things like development, well-being, and the prevention of illness.

Examples include vitamin A, iron, zinc, and tron. For instance, a ron deficiency might inhibit cognitive and motor growth.

The majority of micronutrients may be obtained by consuming lean meats, vegetables, and fruits.

Food Nutrition Recommendations

While there are many guidelines to follow, you should base your diet on experience. This means experimenting with several approaches until you discover one that works for you.

Based on how you eat off someone you want to look like is foolish since everyone has a unique body and genetic composition.

However, there are a few tried-and-true methods that the majority of CrossFitters may follow to increase their fitness improvements over time.

One of them is to adhere to a 40C/30P/30F macronutrient plan.

This indicates that an athlete's caloric intake consists of 40% carbohydrates, 30% protein, and 30% fat.

For instance, if you followed the standard American diet advice of 2,000 calories per day, you would consume 800 calories worth of carbs, 600 calories of protein, and 600 calories of fat. However, most CrossFitters definitely need to eat more than that.

This amounts to 200 grams of carbs, 150 grams of protein, and around 66 grams of fat each day. Then, you may log your food using a macro tracking app like My Macros.

Numerous free macro calculators that account for your age, training age, and weekly physical activity are available online. The If It Fits Your Macros (IIFYM) is sometimes referred to just another diet, although it really serves as the basis for the majority of contemporary monitoring methods.

Weight Loss Diet for Fitness vs. Competitive Weight Loss

Your diet will change depending on your weight loss goals and amount of participation in the sport. One significant difference is that a competitive CrossFit athlete simply has to consume more calories.

Athletes that use competitive CrossFit programming (such as CrossFit Invu or MisFit sports, for instance) train for at least 7.5 hours per week.

Compare that to someone who visits CrossFit 3–4 times a week. Neither is right or wrong, but both situations call for distinct approaches.

Just as a car requires more gas for a longer journey, you'll need to eat more as you exercise. Competing athletes will likely need a lot more carbs than the average gym goer since they are fuel.

What Kind of Crossfit Diet Is There?

In the past, Crust has encouraged a few dietary approaches. Here is a quick introduction to the two most popular diets, the Paleo and the Zone.

Zone Diet The Zone diet uses block counting and a balanced macro split (30/30/40) to ensure that you eat foods that keep you in a healthy "zoe" for performance. It is designed to reduce inflammation and balance hormones.

On the Zone diet, you are theoretically allowed to eat any food, although whole foods are easier to avoid since they are simpler to balance. For further information, see this detailed analysis of the Zone diet.

The Zone Diet has a large variety of dining alternatives and few dietary restrictions, which are its pros. You just need to keep in mind to limit or avoid high glycemic index meals, often known as undesirable foods.

The basic rules for this diet are rather straightforward.

All macronutrients are well-balanced in The Zone diet.

The Proponents of the Zone Diet

If you wish to follow the zone diet to the letter, there is a lot of food measuring required.

It is difficult and involves a lot of preparation, study, reading, and calculating to follow this diet to the letter.

Is the Zone Diet suitable for beginners or is it suited for professionals?

It's simple to start from the beginning if you wish to adhere to the Zone Diet consistently. You may use your body to estimate, or you can use a plate to approximation by putting a third of each (protein, carbohydrates, and fat) on your plate.

Want to see example meal plans for three, four, and five block meals from the CroFt-endorsed Zone diet? Examine this. This fantastic resource offers sample meals for breakfast, lunch, dinner, and snacks.

The Paleo Diet and the Paleo Diet have been intertwined from the very beginning of the sport. One reason for its popularity is because it adheres very closely to Greg Glamour's initial nutritional advice from the 2002 Fitness Journal article "What Is Fitness?" as follows:

Paleo encourages a diet rich in "food a caveman would eat." It has sparked weight loss for many CrossFitters.

But be cautious. You may need to include more carbohydrates in your diet if you exercise often or have an active lifestyle. This Paleo for Athletes book may be able to assist you in finding a balance between competition and healthy eating.

A Paleo diet is a healthy and organic way to eat.

Paleo helps you work out more effectively.

The Paleo diet results in steady blood pressure.

Less body fat was stored.

You get balanced energy from the Paleo diet throughout the day.

smooth skin.

Paleo Cons Paleo may be expensive. Mass-produced meat is more expensive than grass-fed beef and butter.

Avoiding grains and dairy temporarily lowers your energy levels in the early stages since some people experience withdrawal symptoms.

Paleo requires a lot of preparation and cooking at home; it is challenging to eat out when following this diet.

Paleo demands you to learn how to cook or your options will be rather limited. On the Paleo diet, you won't be using packaged or canned foods.

Is Paleo beginner-friendly or only for serious athletes?

If you are currently eating healthily, the Paleo diet is rather simple to adhere to.

If you have previously consumed mostly fast food and processed meals, you will find the Paleo diet to be rather challenging to adhere to.

Unfortunately, success depends more on your cooking prowess than on your degree of athleticism.

If you don't cook and aren't a fan of food prep, you could have more success with a different diet.

The Mediterranean diet is an easier variation of Paleo since it encourages the consumption of healthy fats, fruits, and vegetables from natural sources and discourages the use of packaged, processed, canned, and fast food.

The distinction is that, unlike the Paleo diet, the Mediterranean diet permits dairy, whole grains, and legumes in moderation.

Additionally, the Mediterranean diet does not need tight portion control or calorie tracking, which makes it simpler to adhere to.

The Mediterranean diet might be a good place to start as you make the switch to Paleo.

We Are All Just Getting Started.

From a non-athlete, greetings. Not only a non-athlete, but also someone who had no interest in competing in anything that even somewhat resembled the words "sport" or "group." Or much worse, "partner." This, to my continued enjoyment, occurred before I turned 30 and joined a CrossFit facility. I received my certification as a Level 1 trainer a few years later, which in my younger self would have seemed completely absurd.

Folks, this is what we have. When asked to do one pitiful pull-up for the Presidential Fitness exam, I was only able to hang like a helpless fish on a hook since my best mile in middle school was a 16-minute disaster. In my late 20s, any increase in pulse rate during a brief jog caused my lungs to burn and left a bloody aftertaste in my mouth. After the first session of a "beginners" running class, I came dangerously close to ripping both Achilles tendons, which sidelined me for almost the whole summer. Walking the corporate 5k was a categorical no unless I wanted shin splints to make me useless for a week afterward, and holding my hands above my head to hang a shower curtain to the rod made me see stars and feel like I might pass out. Yoga sounded like a fantastic concept, but it left me feeling very deflated since my muscles were never strong enough to support me in the longer positions. I don't believe I need to provide many more instances to make my argument here: Given that anything that was even vaguely physically active had the same consequence, I wasn't in a great starting position. I came to the realization that I was never going to get well. any one of them. Or so I let myself to think.

Then I began to see folks in their 40s and 50s who, like me, had been sedentary for the most of their life. taking notice. Then it dawned on me. Oh my, this is how it begins and here I was moving in that path. With these folks and their illnesses, it also appeared out of nowhere. starting to feel constantly uncomfortable and stiff, walking up and down stairs, moaning while getting in and out of cars, going to the doctor, and taking medicine. Several medications, naturally for the aches and pains. The inexorable development from pain to knee and hip replacements, followed by the inability to stoop down and get a turkey out of the oven on Thanksgiving, is then what follows. Then followed the falling and breaking of bones after losing equilibrium. Then, for some, WALKING would become a chore. On top of everything else, the continual whining about how miserable they were appeared to dominate every discussion. To be honest, it all felt like a lot of effort. Much more effort is required than just becoming in respectable condition. And let's face it, the cost of all of this appeared to exceed that of a gym membership.

Well, while I wasn't fearful of improving in any of these physical activity-related areas, I was certainly worried of losing my ability to perform them. I made the decision to choose the lesser of two evils and try fitness after a friend of mine who was out of shape raved to me about their really wonderful experience with a nearby CrossFit facility. Again.

I'm hoping that what I learned may help others determine whether or not this kind of training is suited for them, or at the absolute least allow me to express my sincere gratitude to CrossFit for keeping my medical expenses at a zero balance. Despite visiting several gyms around the nation, the CrossFit community has a reputation for being in general frigid and haughty, something I have yet to personally see. The people I have met at these gyms, on the other hand, are the nicest, bravest, and most loving individuals; many of them will become lifelong friends. I've had the privilege of having excellent mentors and coaches from a wide range of backgrounds during my travels. Gymnasts, CrossFit Games winners, Olympic lifting instructors, world-class powerlifting coaches, and both men and women who have served in the military have all trained with me. It is a tremendous and real joy to see how each person's tales intertwine to support others on their travels while working together to achieve challenging tasks.

Everyone brings their own stories and histories with them.

Now for the more challenging, but rewarding, tasks. The questions listed below are ones that you may have wanted to ask but were unsure of who to contact or where to go for reliable answers. By no means am I asserting that my experience is the standard; rather, it is only an honest, first-person narrative for your consideration. It is a pretty succinct overview of the logistical aspect, namely, which I wish I had when I began. I've included a breakdown of many of the many phrases, lingo, and movements as well as some discussion around common problems. In addition, I've included adjustments for several of these motions, if necessary. And I can assure you that it is definitely suggested to alter and do what you can rather than attempting to do what others are doing if you are just getting started. When I first started out, I had all of the aforementioned queries and worries, but I lacked a confidante with whom I could discuss them without feeling self-conscious. It didn't feel great to have to ask a ton of questions about simple matters, and after a workout, I promptly forgot about 99% of the stuff I intended to look up online. But even when I did recall them, I discovered that there was no one point of reference for any of these fundamental concepts. I'm trying to remedy that here. preferably a little.

Frequently Occurring Workout Injuries

We often get so preoccupied with the goals that we forget what it takes to achieve them. Or, at least, that's how I remember my first foray into CrossFit.

There is, without a doubt, always space for development. It doesn't matter whether you've been doing this for years or if you're just starting out and learning the ropes; there is always a chance that you'll hurt yourself.

Of course, individuals who have gotten the hang of it will be less likely to be hurt without warning, but there are a number of other criteria that are crucial to injury avoidance. Inadequate judgment, poor choices, and overall carelessness may all result in tragic events. People who have had the misfortune of being hurt while working out, like as me, will understand just how much it costs. The expense of something does not always indicate what must be done to prevent it from occurring again. Never err on the side of safety.

I didn't like gymnastics or any other kind of athletics when I was little. In reality, I liked the thought of sticking in my own surroundings. I learned, however, that there was a lot of uncertainty between the two sides wanting me to be on their side when my friends and I agreed to get together for a friendly soccer game on a bright day in the middle of the summer. Despite the fact that it wasn't anything major, it did serve as a wake-up call for me. The epiphany caused me to reflect on and assess previous instances when I had been seen as the weak link when it comes to physical pursuits. I was alright as long as I made the choice on my own, but it started to affect me when other people began to assume that I wasn't capable of participating in sports. And with that, an infatuation was created.

I so became determined, albeit I remained as ignorant. The good news is that I've finally been passionate about making this significant shift in my life. After all, it had been a long time coming. The bad news was that I had no notion where to start from earth. Like the ordinary Joe, I went online to look up the simplest of inquiries and see what other internet users had to say. At that point, I learned about high-intensity interval training, or HIIT. The most interesting item I had read about out of everything was that in particular. Later on, I discovered more about CrossFit training, which is a complete training philosophy as well as a kind of HIIT. I went from not being a big fan of exercise to being a walking reference book.

I was more than prepared to use my knowledge in a practical way when the time came. I promptly enrolled in a CrossFit program merely to have a place to practice. My motivation was at an all-time high. I was fired up and believed I could surpass anybody else who shared my objectives.

I injured my lower back after less than two weeks of nonstop exercise.

It turns out that I was so overcome with joy that I totally missed everything that truly mattered in terms of my personal safety. This was a hard blow to me, but it didn't mean that my CrossFit adventure was over. I decided right then and then that it was not the right time to give up on everything that had brought me to that point since I still had a long journey ahead of me. I thus started again, attempting to determine what went wrong the previous time. Like I stated, you either succeed or you fail; my first effort had failed, but I had learned from it.

Regardless of whether you've been there or not, you need to take care of your body just as much as you need to exercise it. Exercise-related injuries are prevalent, but they may be avoided. With the aid of several interrelated aspects, all of which can be grouped under one heading—your well-being— the total risks related to exercise injuries may at the very least be significantly reduced.

WHY TECHNIQUE IS IMPORTANT

Let's start by discussing one of the toughest causes of injury that you could experience: poor technique. Most of the time, you don't realize what you're doing wrong until the effects become apparent. Even athletes sometimes fail to anticipate it since you'll be exhausted after most activities. Contrary to popular belief, fitness is not about how hard you work at it. Instead, you should spend more time becoming more intelligent.

For instance, repeatedly using a joint or muscle when exercising over an extended period of time might cause stress to build up there. When you do an exercise incorrectly, your body does not handle the tension in the manner for which it was intended to do so each time. Imagine it repeating repeatedly until your body's defenses are no longer effective.

This could be prevented. To perfect your technique, all you need is some patience and comprehension. You must ensure that you have a sufficient understanding of what you're getting into before you begin utilizing any equipment or before you just begin exercising without it.

In the ideal situation, a teacher will direct you. It is advisable to avoid the danger if you don't have access to a teacher and you aren't completely confident in what you're doing. You might also ask for advice from others who share your interests, since being around other athletes or more seasoned individuals can help lower the risk of injury. To achieve so, you must first release your ego; if someone notices that you are using poor technique, there is no guilt in enabling them to make the necessary corrections. Remember, taking classes is always a good idea.

Your overall method must also be consistent with the tools you utilize and the attire you don. Equipment may be a possible source of harm if it cannot be relied upon, is too old, or is defective. On the other hand, the way you are dressed might affect how flexible you are throughout your workout. If you're not dressed appropriately for CrossFit training, it will slow you down and impact your technique. There is a reason why specific equipment is made for different kinds of training exercises. Fitness equipment provides your muscles with the best possible operating conditions and speeds up blood flow throughout your body. Additionally, athletic clothing is far more breathable.

You should include pre-workout planning in your strategy as well. A poor training session might result from a poor preparation. The warm-ups that trainers do before to their sessions create the groundwork for the subsequent real business. Warm-ups have been shown to help the blood circulate. Your body's muscles warm up and loosen up as a result of this. On the other hand, jumping right into the action without warming up can not only hinder your performance during the high-intensity workout but also increase your risk of injury since your muscles may be tight. Many times, warm-ups are omitted to save time. Recognize that getting more done in less time doesn't necessarily result in the greatest outcomes.

More is not always better.

CrossFit is more of an art than a workout in my opinion. It is referred to as "the sport of fitness" philosophically. You are able to comprehend, absorb, and live it. If you want to improve, don't anticipate seeing improvements right away. Doing more doesn't necessarily translate into being better than the competition. Some people may find it unexpected, but CrossFit isn't really about speed. Take it one pulse at a time, gradually. Do this until the "new" becomes the "normal." By the time your exercise is through, you can be drenched in sweat, but it in no way ensures a productive session.

Unless, of course, you want to perspire a lot.

When your focus is on gains, you put forth a lot of effort every day. But keep in mind that is one of the most typical errors you may make. Results don't appear right away. Unfortunately, the majority of us lack the patience necessary to deal with that concept. Know when to quit before you do anything else. Physically, the practice of endurance training puts a lot of strain and stress on your body. You have limitations, just like everyone else. While pushing such boundaries can seem inspiring, there are responsible and constructive ways to do so. It's similar to the proverb "Rome wasn't built in a day." Being in the same pattern repeatedly will make you feel frustrated when you don't see results, but try not to allow that aggravation cloud your judgment.

You could be thinking, "What have I got to lose?" What's the response to that query? your wellbeing. It's quite normal to skip one or more days of your exercise schedule. It's not appropriate to make up for it the next day by exerting greater effort. Additionally, avoid being the weekend warrior who rushes through everything rather than taking the time to create a balanced routine. You would be suffering yourself without even realizing it if you lack equilibrium. Even if you may have heard about people becoming overnight successes, athleticism's reasoning just does not support them. In other words, when it's time to quit, stop. If you go on in the belief that nothing negative will occur, don't be shocked when it does.

The problem is that some of us are stronger than others by nature. Some of us believe that our regular exercise days might really help us accomplish more.

Even if you put in twice as much effort as the others, you may still feel good at the end of the day. But exercising unquestionably has limitations, just like anything else that has ever been. Your chance of suffering an injury increases the more you push those limits. Consider your body as a figurative machine to solve the aforementioned conundrum. It is comparable to choosing to drive a car indefinitely until it breaks, at which point the idea of "forever" is no longer applicable. Your body will be forced to give up in some way due to persistently imposed pressure and stress. So, always work harder than you have to but never more so than you ought to.

FAULTY NUTRITION

Diet is important. It is undoubtedly among the most important parts of your body's health. Being well-nourished is incredibly crucial for your general health, even if you don't exercise. It's much more crucial if you're an athlete, and this is a known truth. The rule is straightforward: eat to avoid accidents. You're not necessarily in shape just because you've put in a lot of time at the gym or fitness facility. Speaking from my experience, this was another beginner error I made when I initially began my CrossFit training. The reduction in my performance forced me to recognize the issue, and then the challenge of fixing it presented itself. You should be mindful of what you eat in addition to the physical activity you engage in.

Your muscles break when you exercise, practically regardless of the activity. Know that stinging sensation you get after doing the most push-ups in one set, breaking your personal record? Your body is informing you that your muscles need to be repaired since tissue damage has happened. This is quite typical. Your body actively searches for essential ingredients to aid in the healing process after such an occurrence. It seeks for high-quality protein with more precision. Both before and after the exercise, your body needs to be hydrated and fed throughout the day. You will almost certainly end up losing weight rather than gaining it if you are exercising diligently but are not paying careful attention to what your body requires.

But it doesn't imply you should skip any of the food on the menu. Food is important, but the kind of food your body consumes is more important. You are what you consume, to put it simply. This saying has a lot of meaning, but in the realm of fitness, it is taken literally. After engaging in arduous exercise, you can't expect your body to be in excellent form by downing harmful meals. You may be hurt by eating poorly just as much as by not eating at all. Foods high in sugar and fat are often associated with loss of muscle, bone density, etc. Your body will suffer if it is not properly supported. First of all, if your diet is poor, you'll notice that your exercise performance isn't exactly up to par. Additionally, you run a higher risk of being hurt if you do poorly. A lousy diet cannot be overcome by exercise.

THINGS' MENTAL SIDE

You might get psychologically exhausted after an intense exercise in addition to physically. When opposed to mental weariness, physical exhaustion is simpler to get over. You can find it very difficult to regain motivation once it's gone. Therefore, even if you have all the physical power in the world, your performance will suffer if you are not fully engaged on the task at hand. It's time for a break if you constantly feel lightheaded, exhausted, or simply unable to complete a task. From a safety standpoint, it's far better for you to back off when you're emotionally worn out than to keep going and risk unintentionally hurting yourself.

One of the main reasons for exercise injuries is overtraining. Although you may be exercising on a balanced schedule and taking it easy, it's crucial to keep in mind that not all brains function in the same manner. Exercise is good for you no matter how you do it. However, it is only true if your mind is at ease and focused on what you are doing. Although this is usually true to all athletes, novices who have trouble selecting the right workout are particularly in need of this advice. It's a good idea to vary your routine and add more diversity to your activities. Change is necessary. If you exercise in a constant loop, you'll inevitably become weary and bored and ultimately lose interest in what you're doing.

Your mind must be present at all times if you want to accomplish your goals. You must simultaneously teach your brain to take control of your actions as well as your body. Some extremely significant exercise-related parameters are influenced by your brain. The capacity to withstand, respond, exert, and react are all brain-related abilities. Your brain is in charge of cognitive regulation, which instructs your body on how to react in certain circumstances. Long-term effort might produce uncomfortable circumstances. During intense activities, your mind will cause muscle changes to maintain your body acclimated to your action. The ability of the brain to remain balanced while tired is limited. Inaccurate balance might make injuries more likely. You should constantly pay attention to what your mind is telling you, as a result.

How Can Crossfit Training Benefit You?

The fact that more people are becoming health-conscious is really positive. In fact, a large number of men and women from all over the globe are looking for an edge in the field of health. This is where CrossFit preparation comes into its own, as it is a very effective way to trim your body and boost your wellbeing. Therefore, we should now discover the benefits of CrossFit preparation.

One benefit of CrossFit preparation is that it produces noticeable effects quickly. Typically, all you have to do is eventually apply to begin performing CrossFit preparation. At the conclusion of the preparation, you should be able to tell that your muscle has improved and that your overall wellbeing level has increased. When compared to others who use the customized exercises offered at wellness facilities, you will also notice that your energy has improved. Then once again, you must ensure that you do out the exercise correctly in order to feel its effects in just a short period of time.

In addition to the long list of benefits of CrossFit training, this is also a balanced schedule. It is crucial to make sure your whole body is included while working outside. This is to ensure that you have a physique that is proportioned and very well-toned, as opposed to others who just focus on one certain body part. Because CrossFit preparation uses an all-encompassing approach, you can expect that there are several training styles that will improve the fitness of your whole body.

Wellness enthusiasts often deceive themselves and give up on their schedules on the pretext that they are too exhausted to continue. Due to CrossFit activities, you won't feel worn out. You may explore a selection of workouts referred to as WODs (Workout of the Day) each and every day. In fact, you won't feel tired and you can end up obsessively becoming occupied with your routines, step by step.

Another benefit of CrossFit preparation is that it is moderate. There is no need for you to get special gear later on in order to do the tasks you must. The majority of the exercises in the workout get your body moving with the end objective of achieving a fitter physique. This is not the same as other types of schedules where you are need to purchase your own specialized equipment in order for your activities to be carried out successfully. Clearly, this is one of the benefits of our project that you will like the most.

Beyond the benefits of CrossFit preparation assistance, this kind of preparation is also viable in terms of shaping your own particular physique prior to engaging in any kind of schedule. This prevents your body from feeling any anxiety. Your coaches will initially set up your framework via the presentation of certain preparatory activity schedules before introducing you to another schedule. You won't run into too much problem when you complete the more difficult schedules in the future. When compared to other activity schedules offered by several wellness foundations, this is very different.

These are some of the benefits that you might get by doing CrossFit Preparing. This is perhaps one of the most motivating schedules you may try to follow in order to get the kind of physique you have been longing for. It is crucial that you just put your confidence in experienced prepared specialists or instructors who will manage such preparation if you need to experience the benefits of CrossFit training. This is an immediate consequence of the preparation's particular sort of activity. It is impossible for you to experience the benefits of CrossFit preparing without assessing your abilities and understanding about the system. Hush, how about we move on to the unique activities of CrossFit?

Cross-Training Benefits For Cyclists

What is general education, and how can it work? How does it function?

Your heart is unable to distinguish sports when you participate in any intense activity. This is due to the heart's inability to discern what game you are playing and instead just observing "how hard you are working."

Therefore, you may play just about any intense game and become "for the most part fit." Your leg muscles, on the other hand, need to "explicitly" adapt to the game you are playing. For instance, if you run, your muscles will get used to running. However, since you are jogging instead of riding, your level of "cycling explicit muscle wellness" will significantly decline.

We may thus conclude that general education creates overall wellbeing via playing a variety of games, but be aware that if you play a variety of games consistently, your specific cycling wellness will go. Is teaching everyone in a wide sense counterintuitive?

Maintaining a little amount of riding is the key to successful general education since you don't want to lose all of your previously acquired cycling fitness.

While you establish "general wellness" with your other high-intensity activities, maintaining a few of rides each week is necessary to keep your muscles used to cycling. This is how cross-training is done in an efficient manner.

But if I lose part of my bike fitness, what use is wide education?

It is the perfect time for a mental vacation if you've spent the whole summer participating in cyclosportives, traveling, or just riding your bike nonstop.

Building up slowly in this way by needing some time away from year-round riding suggests that you will return fit and renewed. When you're ready, be prepared to emphasize your cycle preparation more. Ideally, you wouldn't want to maintain the same level of wellbeing throughout the whole year. Instead, you should improve your wellness to a couple of tops over the cycling summer, not during the holidays.

Additionally, educating yourself widely may help you strengthen your bones and muscles that you don't utilize for riding. For instance, weight-bearing activities like jogging, walking, climbing, and gym training may help strengthen your bones and prevent osteoporosis. More bikers, especially women, should be aware of these benefits.

Cross-country skiing, swimming, trail jogging, snowshoeing, inline skating, and paddling are a few more examples of high-intensity sports you could take into consideration. If you've been out and about in the late spring, think about going hiking in the mountains. You'll spend time in the outdoors, build strong legs, and avoid road traffic.

Be aware that there is a learning curve with these activities, so start off slowly as your body gets used to the new workout. The main takeaway from this is that cross-training enables you to be totally fit and refreshed over the course of a few months whereas individuals who have been riding their bikes all winter will most likely be exhibiting indications of fatigue and ennui.

Enjoy your holiday, enjoy some new games, and look forward to the local greatest rides in a year when the weather is at its best and you're feeling good.

Why Do It That Way: The Ins And Outs:

The ultimate crossfit training guide: why do people do crossfit? Well, sometimes people just want to feel good about themselves, therefore in order to do this, they subject themselves to grueling workouts. things that often cause them to pass out and may leave them hurting for days afterwards.

Sound enjoyable? No, I don't believe so. Fortunately, this is not all that crafting is about. Yes, some individuals work out really hard, and these are the ones who finally get strong and fit enough to participate in events like the CrossFit Games.

For the average person, however, corruption is as difficult as you would want it to be. Be my guess if you want to send yourself to hell and back. However, if you want to have a somewhat comfortable yet challenging work season, then corruption is ideal.

There are a number of benefits associated with crossfit, including (but by no means limited to!)

• It will assist you in losing weight if you need to.

If you struggle with getting to the gym on your own, it might help you remain motivated to work out. It's a fantastic way to maintain physical and mental health.

• You'll meet kind, like-minded people, and who knows—you could even make new long-term friends!

However, there is a little issue that, for some of us, detracts from the beauty of craftsmanship: It is often quite expensive. Since many people cannot afford it, they decide not to join a commercial gym. If that's the case, don't try since there's a solution!

Crossfit workouts that are free for students (and those who can't afford gyms):

Crossfit workouts for free at home are possible! Although you may not have the equipment and exercise machines required to execute every cross-fit workout, you will discover that you can really do the majority of things.

This is due to the fact that a large portion of crossfit revolves on exercises that use your natural body weight to provide stability for your muscles to move around. This means that everyone and anybody can do various crossfit routines, regardless of where they live or how poor they are.

There are numerous crossfit routine examples on the internet, and I've even included a few of my favorites a little bit further in the article. Simply choose your exercises, watch a few videos on how to do them, and presto, you have your very own workout regimen that can be completed in the comfort of your own living room!

How Much Is Crossfit?

As previously said, corruption, regrettably, has a tendency to be rather expensive. But if you join a high-quality gym, you definitely get what you pay for. Many head coaches, assistant coaches, as well as simple helpers are present at most commercial gyms to ensure that you get the most out of your exercise.

If you're unsure about whether you can afford the expense of CrossFit, consider this: It is much less expensive than hiring your own personal trainer and is unquestionably less expensive than scheduling one-on-one sessions a couple times per week with this personal trainer.

If you're still unsure, I'd suggest visiting a crossfit gym to find out what all the fuss is about. Most gyms let you to have one or two trials before you must join up, so it would be quite wise of you to take advantage of this.

Does corruption work?

To make it brief and straightforward, yes, coding works. It is a quick and effective way to develop your body and get a high level of general fitness.

However, it's crucial to remember that success is not the goal if you're attempting to train for a certain activity or a specific ability, like endurance jogging. In these situations, you are going to do far better finding a coach who is familiar with the skill or sport you are training for and concentrating on exercises that will improve it.

Is it suitable for me?

Many individuals, in my humble opinion, are tremendously resentful of corruption. There are also:

Freaks and freaks: The goal of cruelty is to push the human body to and over its limits. This makes it the ideal sport for fitness fanatics and those who sometimes appreciate a little (or a lot) of pain. I'm not lying; I've seen people push themselves so hard to battle their fatigue that they leave or spend the next 10 minutes leaving the room.

Athletes and aspiring athletes - Aspiring athletes who are used to the camaraderie and competitiveness seen in professional or semi-professional sports are often well-suited to progress.
People who like working with and around other people - Crossfit is for you if you like working out in groups or with your friends. Working with others may be a great way to boost your drive and push yourself to reach your next goal, even if it sometimes means sacrificing a little bit of privacy and making yourself seem like a Turk.

People seeking assistance or who are new to training - Crossfit at home is one alternative, but it lacks the support and sense of community that you'll get in a crossfit facility. If you lack confidence, are a little uncertain of yourself, and sometimes struggle to stay motivated, then coaching is probably for you.

How can I become a corrupter?

What does the word "crofit" mean? And I don't mean "what is craft," but rather, "what does it mean to be a crafter"? Crossfit often has a positive impact on a person's life. It may result in extensive lifestyle adjustments, often for the better. For instance, a really dedicated crossfitter would give up alcohol and focus on eating a completely healthy, balanced diet.

Getting into craft is as simple as walking up to a craft gym and asking to have a try. Try another gym if they don't welcome you with open arms. Crossfit is about community and camaraderie, thus an unfriendly gym won't be enjoyable!

Don't be discouraged by bulky weights or challenging-looking exercises; you won't be the only beginner at the gym.

How Does Crossfit Work?

Every craft gym often has its own identity and brand name. In the gym, as you get to know the trainers and coaches, you'll start to feel like a member of the CrossFit family. I promise you that.

Your results are recorded when you engage in craft projects. Most crossfit clubs upload these results to the internet so that you may compare your performance to that of others in your gym, your city, and even the best in the whole world. This implies that you always have something to aim towards and that you can easily keep track of your progress.

Do you play a competitive sport?
Absolutely, yes! A quick glance at the World Championship schedule reveals a wide variety of professional and semi-professional competitions. Although the majority of us will probably never reach

that level, it is still good to know that it is feasible.

The even more exciting aspect about crossfit, especially if you compete, is that you can compare your results to those of practically every other athlete in the world (or at the very least in your country). The majority of crossfit gyms have a recording system that involves capturing your crossfit results and putting them into an online database. This database allows you to keep track of your development and compare your outcomes to those of other crossfitters across the globe.

The F**king Games

The CrossFit Games are a competition where some of the world's most well-rounded athletes unite to compete for the title of Fittest Man (or Woman) on Earth Crew.

The games were developed to fill a void. "There was no other genuine fitness test. All other athletic events, from Ironman triathlons to the NFL, failed to accurately assess athletes' fitness. Even decathlons, which assessed a very wide range of abilities, had important elements of physical fitness.

The Games are divided into three phases rather than being held as a single event. The OPEN, a five-week competition with five workouts that takes place in winter at CrossFit affiliates and general gyms all around the globe, is the first stage.

The best competitors from 18 different international areas qualify for the CrossFit Regionals stage of the tournament once the Open is over. The 18 international regions compete against one another at Regionals in one of nine events. The winners are then eligible for berths in the Cross Games.

By the time the CrossFit Games begin, the field has been reduced from hundreds of thousands of athletes in the Open to the top 40 men, 40 women, 40 teams, 80 youths, and 240 judges, who all compete to determine who is the fittest person on Earth.

What tools do I need for crafting?

If you go to a true fitness center, you just need the standard gym essentials (shoes, a water bottle, a towel, and sometimes a stopwatch). However, if you want to start doing more cardio exercises at home, you will need to invest in additional equipment.

Some great items to invest in for use in your own home are free weights (medical balls and kettlebells), a yoga mat, exercise bands, and some kind of chin-up and dip bar.

Will Clutter Help You Lose Weight?
Yes. Naturally, it will. If you burn more calories than you consume, you will lose weight in any activity. And making food involves a lot of effort.

A study that was published in the International Journal of Sports and Exercise Medicine found that 27. Normal CrossFit athletes (not the competitors you see at the Games) were randomized to either train CrossFit for 6 weeks while restricted to a low-carb keto diet or to train CrossFit for 6 weeks while adhering to their regular diet. They discovered that those who paired butter with a ketogenic diet significantly decreased weight, body fat percentage, and body mass.

Weight, body fat percentage, and fat mass dramatically decreased in those who combined CrossFit with the keto diet.

But don't let that study lead you to believe that in order to experience the benefits of CroFt, you must adopt the keto diet. Remember that CrossFit recommends a balanced diet, or, in other words, eating "meat and vegetables, nuts and seeds, some fruit, little starch, and no sugar."

How Much Muscle Can You Develop Through CrossFit?

Strength training expert Mark Rippetoe claims that "CrossFit has provided more people with access to bars and the motivation to lift them than any other single factor in the past hundred years."

Obviously, if you pick up a barbell often enough, you'll develop muscle, but is it possible to develop more muscle via

CrossFit than through a conventional bodybuilding regimen?

A Comprehensive Guide To Bodybuilding

The results of a research published in the International Journal of Sports Physical Therapy comparing the benefits of functional and conventional strength training in men revealed "no differences in improvement between the training protocol."

It doesn't really matter whether you pick up a barbell in a traditional gym or in a Fit Box if you're trying to build muscle. You can create a lot in both.

However, if you're concerned that all of that conditional work in CroFt would harm your earnings, don't be; it won't. Studies carried out at the Department of Health Sciences in Mid Sweden Research has shown that adding cardio to a leg-strengthening program really increased muscle size rather than decreased it.

Craft tips and tricks:

Going down to a brand-new fitness facility and just giving it a go isn't always as simple as it sounds. We have created a collection of excellent tips and methods that will help you start your entrepreneurial journey:

Check out a few gyms before joining one:

Choosing a crossfit gym is analogous to choosing a family since they are all striving for the same or similar goals as you are. Therefore, choosing a good fitness facility where you feel welcomed and where everyone is friendly is crucial.

Most commercial gyms provide the first session for free, so you should probably take advantage of this. Try out many gyms in your area before choosing on one, and remember that even if you choose one but later decide that you don't like it, you can really switch gyms rather quickly.

Contrary to what many people believe, success is all about enjoying yourself and improving the quality of your life. If you only seem to have time for one workout session each week, that is definitely OK. There is no need to push yourself above your point of comfort since doing so will decrease your pleasure and take away from the benefits of profit.

Go at your own pace while exercising: If you really want to see improvements in your health and fitness, you'll need to be prepared to make some adjustments in your lifestyle. It is entirely up to you whether this entails a whole diet overhaul or just getting up an hour earlier so that you have enough time to go to the gym. Just be aware that fitness is a way of life, not something that happens at the gym.

The most important thing is to get there, challenge yourself, and meet new people:

After all, the primary reason why corruption has spread so widely around the world is due to its social aspect. So go ahead and do it: go outside, have fun, and discover the benefits of what we affectionately refer to as crossfit!

Food That Is Ideal For Crossfitters

These foods put your body in an optimal, supercharged condition that will have you spinning your tires in no time! Check them out, and then continue reading to find out what to avoid.

1.Lentils

"Cro-Fitters need to keep their protein intake around 30 percent of their daily calories—and minimally add a whopping nine grams of protein per half cup to your meal, with loads of fiber," advises Cat Smiley, CPT, author of The Plant-Friendly Diet and proprietor of Whistler Fitness Vacations, a weight loss retreat in British Columbia, Canada.

Extremely adaptable, use them in omelets, chili dishes, and more.

2. Banana and whipping cream smoothie

"Post-workout, you need to refuel and optimize recovery by replenishing your glycogen stores and protein for tissue repair. Your body desires both quickly digesting carbs, such as those found in fruits and baked goods, and quickly and easily absorbable proteins, such as whey, according to MS, RD registered dietitian and founder of The WellNecessities. Just make sure your wheat protein powder is pure and does not include a laundry list of fillers and chemicals.

3. Conut oil

You may have spent money on a container of the product to have smoother skin and shinier hair, but adding it to your diet is a CrossFitter's absolute must-do: "Coconut oil is an excellent source of fuel for workouts. Peggy Kotokoulos, RHN, nutritionist and author of Kitchen Cures, explains that while it is a heated fat, the medium-chain fatty acids in it make it quickly absorbable by the small intestine (without requiring the complete digestion process).

This means that it gives off more energy faster than any other fat. The liver transforms fat into an instant energy source, just as it would do with carbs, but it's sugar- and carbohydrate-free! Try a tablespoon of it before to working out, and you'll be astounded at the energy and endurance it offers.

Nutty and Seedy

"Nuts and seeds are packed with nutrients and omega-3 fatty acids, which will fuel your recovery after an intense CrossFit WOD," suggests Karla Willam, an enthusiastic CrossFitter and owner of South Carolina's Healthy Kitchen, a retreat and wellness center for weight loss.

Since nuts and seeds are high in calories, they make a delicious on-the-go snack or addition to a filling smoothie.

Five. Sweet potatoes

The Instagram stream of this tubercular vegetable may have calmed down after the fall, but there are still plenty of reasons to seek for this food source of power: Your body need functional carbohydrates for an energy boost. Your body uses the glucose stored in your muscles (and liver) as energy to carry you through your workday. Glycogen is stored in your muscles via the digestion of carbohydrates.

"One of the best ways to fuel this is with sweet potatoes, which are complex carbohydrates that are slowly released and will keep you going during your workout. Sweet potatoes provide consistent, steady energy levels by balancing blood sugar levels. They are also rich in B6, which counteracts the physical effects of stress that the body experiences after a workout, and rich in antioxidant vitamin V. Beta-carotene and vitamin C help to repair free radical damage brought on by working exercise. Start salivating over these sweet potato dishes right now.

6. Banana and almond butty

Not in the mood to go to Smoothe-ville, exactly? It's okay. This nutrient-dense snack is beneficial for CrossFitters: "If you do CrossFit, your ideal snack will be a blend of carbohydrates, protein, and a small amount of healthy fat."The banana in this recipe is crucial since it is a great source of potassium, which is required to help the heart and skeletal muscles flex and contract during your work out.

7.Eggs

"Eggs are a superior food for gluten eaters since they are packed with protien, vitamin B, and healthy fats. A single egg has 7 to 10 grams of protein. Starting the day with a few eggs boosts your daily protein budget.

8.Brown Rice

"Brown rice is healthier for you than white rice since it hasn't been refined and bleached to remove nutrients. It is also easily digested and less likely to result in bloating and rises in blood pressure. Make a large quantity at the start of the week and use with various proteins, vegetables, and sauces.

9. Nut butter

Welcome to Destination: Dream Food. The potential for this tasty spread is endless.Put a few teaspoons of almond butter in your favorite latte or use it as a spread or dip. Almond butter has roughly four grams of protein and eight grams of fat per tablespoon. We all know that protein is king for those who are overweight, but don't forget the crucial role that fat plays: "Fat is important for fat as well because it's yet another fantastic source of long-lasting energy."

10.Oatmeal

Oatmeal is a popular morning food that is stylish when prepared as overnight oats. Though it's a must-have for cake eaters as well: "Oatmeal is a great pre- or post-workout food as it delivers carbohydrates to the body efficiently without needless supplications," says Hayim. It also seems to be exceptional for muscle recovery.

Cross-Training Features And Components.

Weightlifting

It is now essential to maintain a healthy, robust physique. This clearly well-known pattern has helped people pay greater attention to their true selves and to the value of good health.

People now spend a lot of money on weightlifting equipment to get the real physique they have always desired.

Both men and women have realized that weightlifting would not only improve their physical health but also their appearance and how the rest of the world perceives them. People are looking for the best techniques to get rid of excess body fat and get the perfect body shape.

They put a lot of time, effort, and money into shaping their bodies and living better lives. Weightlifting regimens may also protect people against a wide range of illnesses by strengthening and improving the heart, lungs, and liver as well as their brains.

An individual with devotion may finally achieve the optimal body type and physical health by doing weightlifting in the proper way, at the right intensity, and while adhering to all safety precautions and measures.

People often join gym facilities where they are provided with a broad variety of professional weight lifting equipment to help them build their bodies in order to get their desired real look. Additionally, coaches are available to assist people in carrying out the proper tasks in the proper manner so that their workout program produces the greatest and most effective outcomes.

The trainers provide their professional judgment so that the person learns correct procedures and ensures that overexertion does not occur. The gym has equipment like weights, heavy balls, treadmills, cycles, etc. that people may use depending on their exercise routine.

Some people, however, are unable to join a gym and develop the physique they find perfect owing to their hectic job schedules and other circumstances. In such circumstances, customers may purchase the necessary equipment from a variety of retail establishments that are reachable anywhere.

Make sure you see a doctor and a nutritionist before beginning a weightlifting program. This will help you plan a proper workout regimen that will be helpful in correctly strengthening and nurturing your physique. You will get the physique you normally want if you use legal methods, exhibit caution, and maintain your workout schedule.

Gymnastics

If you like doing aerobatics, you should be somewhat knowledgeable about the equipment you will use to tumble. Being acquainted with the general courses and standard equipment is a terrific idea since this is a topic that is especially excellent.

The equilibrium pillar is one such item of hardware. Although there are several little deviations from this, the shaft itself is somewhat identical. They are available in lengths of 8' or 10', and they are a few inches broad. An fitness facility will include a pillar that protrudes only a few inches above the ground for beginners. For a lot of folks, even and lopsided bars are just another noticeable piece of hardware. Although these pieces of equipment are different, the skills needed to use them are comparable.

Vaulting equipment is important, but since it is seldom the focus of attention, it often gets overlooked without much of a problem. However, there are several varieties of vaulting gear. The springboard is the most well-known kind. Various types of aerobatic equipment are used in tandem with vaulting components.

Another important piece of gear that is usually overlooked is landing pads. Gymnasts might truly suffer injury during a regular practice without the proper mats. The mats must be strong enough to let the participant nail their finish while also being sensitive enough to absorb the impact of their landing.

Two of three common types of acrobatic equipment are rings and equal bars. These are both used mostly by males, despite the fact that they are both Olympic sports. For both adults and children, almost every kind of acrobatic equipment is available. Both the elements and the safety measures will be special. The padding on the equipment for children will be substantially greater.

Any acrobat should possess exceptional practical dexterity and the ability to assess how much effort they are putting into a maneuver. They must dirty their turn or overshoot their impression if they strain themselves too much. They will miss the target if they put forth insufficient effort. Any situation has the potential to result in a bodily problem. It should always be kept in mind that tumbling is difficult to accomplish correctly, and anybody trying to use any acrobatic equipment without the proper training risks significant injury. Even seasoned gymnasts shouldn't do exercises without a spotter.

Cardio

Cardiovascular workouts are done to strengthen and build your heart, train your lungs, and improve your circulation, blood flow, and breathing capacity. Together, these components form the "framework" of your cardiovascular system. Therefore, the primary benefit of cardio training is to further enhance your body's cardiovascular system by getting it ready to function more effectively.

What aerobic activity is most effective?

The most clear answer is usually the one you'll find most difficult to believe when you hear it. In essence, the finest aerobic workout you will ever do in your life is the one you already do! What we're trying to convey is that you shouldn't spend a lot of time experimenting with every new cardio program or cardio exercise that is on the market. Your energy would be better spent if you actually DID the exercise.

What aerobic exercises are best performed at home?

Undoubtedly, going for a simple stroll is one of the least taxing ways to engage in a good cardio workout. But bear in mind to walk quickly enough to maintain an elevated heart rate! You might perhaps go for a run as an alternative. If you are sufficiently lucky to come upon a pool, you may take a dive; just make sure you are swimming laps!

Now, there are many of workouts you might perform indoors if the weather is bad. Whatever the case, they often call for a certain piece of equipment. Treadmills and activity bikes are usually the most well-known goods since they are remarkable devices that don't take up a lot of room.

What equipment works best for aerobic exercises?

You don't need to worry with any special apparatus to get into cardiovascular fitness, as we recently looked at. However, given that this website is dedicated to gym equipment, we would be remiss if we neglected to include some of the best cardio devices.

Can Beginners Do Crossfit

This program is intended for universal use, making it the ideal application for any committed individual regardless of experience. We have used the same procedures for elderly individuals with heart problems who have been removed from television shows for one month. We scale load and intensity; we don't change programs." That means that every day, a specific exercise is prescribed for everyone who attends CrossFit.

Instead than having separate workouts for older women and hard-core athletes, there is one program available every day that is completely scalable based on your skill. For instance, if the exercise calls for barbell squats with 135 pounds but you can only do squats with the bar (45 pounds), that is where you will begin. A similar movement will be substituted if you are injured and unable to do the exercise at all, and if the number of repetitions is too high for your current level of fitness, it will be lowered. As you get stronger and more skilled, you'll eventually execute the tasks as they are described. CrossFit is ideal for a select few types of individuals, even though it may be for everyone:

Weight training beginners - CrossFit is a terrific place for you to start if you've never worked out with weights before (or if you've just worked out on machines) provided you have a decent routine, which I'll go into in a moment. You will be taught how to do all of the crucial lifts in a setting that is very encouraging and judgment-free. You could even discover that, gasp, you like weight training.

People seeking community and support This is what draws me to CrossFit: Every CrossFit facility has a strong sense of community. You are a person who needs help, not just something they can use as payment for membership. When Nerd Fitness clubs start opening (don't think it won't happen!), I'll be drawing a lot of inspiration from CF in terms of how the members are so kind and accepting of one another.

Fitness fanatics are those people you know who like working out every day and feel as if something is happening if they don't. Because of the way CroF is set up, you are working with regular consistency. The typical protocol is three days on and one day off, although many CrossFitters find themselves in the gym more regularly. It's compulsive.

I mean it in the nicest manner imaginable, Masochist. CrossFit often rewards participants for completing workouts in the shortest amount of time possible. This means that you will often find yourself in circumstances where you are using all of your effort to complete a task, depleting yourself, and forcing yourself to push through the fight.

Former athletes: CrossFit has competition, camaraderie, and teamwork built right in. Most workouts have a time component to them, where you must either do a certain number of repetitions of exercises in a specific amount of time, or the time is fixed, and you must determine how many repetitions of an exercise you are capable of performing. You get to compete with classmates and check your results online against the best CrossFit athletes in the world. Even an international competition exists for those who become really dedicated. There are a few individuals for whom I do not believe that CrFt would be as beneficial, although this does not imply that they would not like it:

Specialists - CrossFit takes pride in not specializing, thus anybody trying to specialize (like a powerlifter) won't get the best results by adhering to the standard CrossFit workout schedule. Your focus should be on that activity if you wish to excel at it.

Sport-specific athletes - Similar to the experts, if you are an athlete practicing for a competition, you would be better suited hiring a coach who is skilled at generating outstanding results out of athletes in your particular sport. Every sport has unique movements that call for certain sorts of muscle strength. CroFt gets you ready for anything, but it won't improve your specific sport skills unless you're working on them. Many athletes opt to mix CrossFit with sport-specific exercises (such as CrossFit Football) in their off-season for conditioning, although it is entirely up to each athlete's personal preference.

Solo exercisers - Some people, like myself, like to exercise alone; I train alone every day. CrFt is group training, thus you won't have the chance to do your work on your lonesome.

How dangerous is the truth?

CrossFit may be dangerous in the wrong circumstances, with the wrong instructors, and for someone with the incorrect attitude:

During a CrossFit workout, you're often instructed to complete a certain number of strength training or endurance exercises as quickly as possible, or to complete as many repetitions as you can in a certain period of time.

For this reason, it's quite simple to compromise form in exchange for completing the exercise more quickly. You're in trouble if no one is teasing you or telling you to maintain your proper form.

When it comes to strength training, using improper form—especially at high speeds with big weights—is the quickest way to sustain a catastrophic injury.

Things like these happen often if a CrossFit gym is operated by inexperienced and untested coaches, which is unquestionably the case.

Crème draws a certain kind of person, notably those who push themselves to the point where they injure themselves physically. Ask any crocheter whether they have ever encountered "Pukey the Clown," and they will likely answer in the affirmative.

Due to the nature of competition, the motivating environment, and people's drive to succeed, many participants in competitive sports often push themselves over their own limits (which may be beneficial)...However, they often push themselves too far.

An very serious medical condition called rhabdomyolysis may occur in certain extreme circumstances with a very little amount of carbohydrates (or similar types of exercise programs).

People who push themselves too hard, too fast, or both damage their kidneys by releasing their muscle fibers into the circulation.

Some people at Crunch refer to this as "Uncle Rahbdo," even though it's neither amusing or enjoyable.

This often happens to former athletes who haven't worked out in a while and return to attempt to prove something, but wind up training harder than their bodies can manage.

So, just as with any activity, there may be some who want to push themselves too far, too hard, too quickly, and too often.

Unfortunately, due to the nature of cocaine (where this behavior may be encouraged and encouraged by the wrong cocaine), if you don't know when to stop or have a cocaine that will tell you when to stop, you might wind up in some serious trouble. There are problems that tend to affect individuals more than the CrossFit system as a whole, yet it is the nature of CrossFit that draws these people in and motivates them to act dangerously.

Why Are You Being So Expensive?

CroFt offers group classes. There is a coach conducting the session, unlike a typical gym where hundreds of people drop by, use the elliptical for 20 minutes, and go.

Yes, group classes are all that are offered at most Crutchfield gyms. Some commercial gyms are open from 5 am to 11 pm, but not many are, unlike your local commercial gym.

What a kooky pull-uup
A knuckle pull-up is a kind of pull-up in which you swing your body and drive your hips and posterior to the bar. Because it's not intended to be the same workout as a dead-hang pull-up, it is not cheating. Some jobs need a dead-hang pull-up, and in those, you wouldn't be allowed to stop.